SHEA BUTTER

The Nourishing Properties of Africa's Best-Kept Natural Beauty Secret

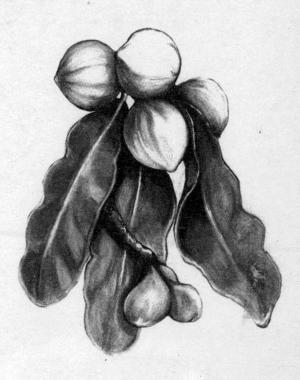

By W.G. Goreja

AMAZING HERBS PRESS
New York, NY

Note: The information in this book is for educational purposes only and is not meant to be a replacement for medical advice, nor is it intended for use in the diagnosis, treatment, cure, or prevention of any illnesses, diseases, or conditions. The authors, publishers, distributors, and owners accept no liability for such use. Anyone suffering from a serious condition should seek the advice of a qualified medical professional.

Amazing Herbs Press
545 Eighth Avenue, Ste. 401
New York, NY 10018
www.AmazingHerbsPress.com

ISBN 0-9742962-5-2

Printed in the United States of America

Table of Contents

Introduction

If shea butter is not *the* most nourishing and moisturizing natural product on the market, it is certainly one of them. Shea not only provides unequalled skin moisturizing, it is clinically proven to heal skin and reduce inflammation. It's a wonderful anti-aging product, and it prevents and then protects against stretch marks during and after pregnancy, after which its usefulness continues as a key baby-care product.

The person who introduced shea to Europe (where it has been used ever since) was the great Scots explorer, Mungo Park (1771-1805). Park was the first European to venture up the Gambia River at the end of the 18th century. He wrote extensively about how native Africans used shea. The following is an excerpt from his book *Travels in the Interior of Africa*,[1] an account of his travels through the then largely undiscovered Dark Continent:

> *They supply the inhabitants of the maritime districts with native iron, sweet-smelling gums, frankincense, and a commodity called shea-toulou, which, literally translated, signifies tree-butter. This commodity is extracted from the kernel of a nut by boiling the nut in water...the extract has the consistency and appearance of butter; and is an*

admirable substitute for it. It is an important staple in the food of the natives and therefore the demand for it is great...the people were everywhere employed in collecting the fruit of the shea trees. These trees grow in great abundance all over this part of Bambarra. They are not planted by the natives, but are found growing naturally in the woods; and in clearing woodland for cultivation; every tree is cut down but the shea. The tree itself very much resembles the American oak; and the fruit, from the kernel of which, being first dried in the sun, the butter is prepared by boiling the kernel in water, has somewhat the appearance of a Spanish olive. The kernel is enveloped in a sweet pulp, under a thin green rind. The butter produced from it, besides the advantage of its keeping the whole year without salt, is whiter, firmer, and, to my palate, of a richer flavor than the best butter I ever tasted made from cow's milk. The growth and preparation of this commodity seem to be among the first object of African industry in Bambarra and the neighboring states; and it constitutes a main article of their inland commerce.

Chapter 1
Description

Belying the way shea adds beauty to our skin, the shea tree appears dry and gnarled, dressed with leathery leaves. A member of the *Sapotaceae* family, native only to the savannah regions of the Sudan, these particular trees resist plantation-based cultivation. Instead, the trees thrive in the ever-receding rain forests and jungles that stretch from Cameroon to Senegal, the Ivory Coast, Nigeria, Togo, Benin, Mali, Niger, and Burkina Faso. This unusual tree grows only 10 to 15 meters high and does not even flower until it is 20 years old. In fact, shea trees only reach maximum productive capacity at the age of 50 years and then remain fully productive for more than a century.

The green, plum-shaped fruits of the shea tree, which become brown when they ripen, can achieve a diameter of about 4 cm. With a fat content of 50%, the nuts and seeds within are a precious source of fat and oil and are used in many ways in their African homeland. It is from these seeds that shea butter is derived.

Chapter 2
Common Names

Known as *karité* in Wolof and as *kare* or *kolo* in Peuhl, the English name shea is derived from the word *se*, used by the indigenous Bambaras peoples of Central Africa. Other common names are *shétoulou* ("tree butter") in the Senegalese language and *ghariti* in the Malian language. The genus name means "butter seed." The tree is also known to science as *Vitellaria paradoxa* and *Butyrospermum parkii*. According to Delta (a botanical reference book), which lists both genuses, the reasons for the splitting of the family *Sapotaceae* into these two genuses are unclear. The Latin name *Butyrospermum parkii* takes the extra tag of "parkii" in honor of Mungo Park.

Chapter 3
Historical Use of Shea Butter

Africa's long relationship with shea butter is both intimate and diverse. In the wooded savannah between Senegal and Nigeria, history and culture are completely enmeshed with the shea tree and its butter.

Accounts from as early as Cleopatra's Egypt speak of caravans bearing clay jars of valuable shea butter for cosmetic use. The funeral beds of early kings were carved in the noble wood of old shea trees. Shea butter has always been a staple of African pharmacology. As mentioned, Mungo Park wrote of the importance of shea butter in everyday life for many of the tribes in Africa. Many other great travelers have recorded their observations about Africa's culture and its use of shea butter. Ibn Batouta was a historian and ambassador whom the Moroccan Sultan entrusted with a diplomatic mission to the court of Mali. Traveling through West Africa in 1348, he described the various uses of shea butter.

Shea butter's amazing skin-care and healing properties were first harnessed thousands of years ago. The history of shea as a precious commodity can be traced back to ancient Egypt, where shea butter was and continues to be used to protect the skin and hair against the fierce sun and the hot dry winds of the African deserts and savannah. The first clues to the anti-inflammatory properties of shea butter came from its documented use as a treatment for rheumatism within traditional African medicine systems. Local healers have also used shea butter to relieve "inflammation of the nostrils" and nasal congestion. Modern research has confirmed shea's effectiveness in this arena.

The traditional applications of shea beyond external use on the visible skin attest to its powerful healing effects. Shea butter is also used for soothing and accelerating healing after circumcision. Also, in the upper river division of The Gambia, a region with a terribly high infant mortality rate (27%), statistics show that the application of shea butter to the baby's umbilical cord stump imparts a recognized protective factor that enhances survival by preventing infection.[2]

Another interesting traditional application of shea butter in West Africa is as an effective insect repellent. Simulium parasitic infection remains a major nuisance in Africa, particularly throughout the forest regions and the fertile valleys of the savannah. The larvae of this organism, which are contracted though bites from the adult black fly, cause severe discomfort and seriously degrade one's quality of life.

Crèmes and lotions containing shea butter have been found to be an effective, affordable, and practical means for individual protection against Simulium infection.[3]

Used in combination with citrus juices such as lime, shea butter is a wonderful antiperspirant and helps reduce associated body odor. Shea butter is also traditionally employed for the relief of rheumatism and muscle and joint pain. This amazing moisturizer has even been used on animals, particularly dogs in Africa, as a moisturizer to protect their skin and their paws from the effects of sand and salt.

Pregnant African women cover their swelling abdomens with shea butter to prevent stretch marks; after birth, the women massage their babies from head to toe with it. In the Beng tribe of the Ivory Coast, mothers rub shea butter over their babies' skin after bathing them to make the children's skin glow. In northeast Ghana, delivering women commonly sit or squat over basins of warm water and shea oil to ease the pains of birth.

Considered sacred and a vessel of mystical power in its homeland, the shea tree is respected and revered. The time of harvest, when the fruits that yield the butter-producing seeds are gathered, is part of an ancient native ritual called *Begu*, the start of which is marked by a wonderful festival wherein people make drink offerings to the gods and, at the festival's high point, a priest slaughters a chicken beneath an ebony tree. According to the tradition of *Begu*, only women are allowed to collect the fruits of this sacred tree. Men are forbidden to lay a hand on the tree or its fruit.

As a versatile source of oil, shea butter is also used to make lamp oil, heating oil, and soap. Shea is also an important source of cholesterol-fighting cooking oil and hardened fat.

Shea oil is an essential ingredient in African cuisine. It is the most desired oil for food preparation and becomes the base of many soups and condiments. Combined with millet flour, water, and different spices, it is used in beverages at weddings, funerals, and work parties. The fat from the first seasonally harvested nuts of the shea tree is used in a traditional dish of brown beans eaten by the village community during Begu.

Chapter 4
Methods of Extraction

Collected shea tree nuts are sun-dried and shelled or cracked by hand with a stone or wooden mallet. If the location is convenient, the nuts may be brought to a gas, diesel, or electric grinding mill; otherwise, the kernels are pounded in wooden or stone mortars to a coarse meal (a cold-press procedure) that can be processed in various ways. One way is to boil the kernels according to an ancient recipe to produce a butter-like mass.

Once the nuts have been reduced to a fine paste, water is added and the paste is rapidly mixed to beat air into it, similar to way whipped cream is made. Warm water is then added to the mixture to dissolve the fat, and the mixture is then whipped again. At this point, cool water sprinkled over the resulting compounds causes the separated fat to harden. This procedure is repeated until a heavy white mass, which is not quite solid and not quite liquid, is slowly extracted. This white mass or suspension must then be drained, boiled, and filtered and left to sit in the sun to cure.

Other refining methods utilize the bleaching properties of the hot, dry earth and involve steaming the meal to deodorize the

shea butter, which helps remove its characteristic earthy odor.
The color of the resulting shea butter can range from white to
golden yellow and, if the butter is properly dried and stored,
can last for several years. Efficient extraction requires deep
knowledge and years of experience. Industrialized modern
methods of extraction often utilize various solvents such as
hexane. One of the negative aspects of this type of extraction
is that it reduces the total availability of certain fractions such
as tocopherol (vitamin E), which affects the stability of the
finished product by reducing its antioxidant capability, making
it prone to rancidity .

Chapter 5
Why Rancidity Equals Poor Quality

At room temperature, premium shea butter is a soft, uniformly beige, creamy solid that readily melts in the hands and is quickly absorbed by the skin. When left in a hot room or near a heat source, shea butter readily melts, just as any butter does. At room temperature, shea butter spreads as easily as soft butter or margarine. Unaltered shea butter has no perfume fragrance.

If your shea butter lacks the characteristic smell and color and does not spread like butter, it is probably of low quality. Rancidity results directly from the oxidation of the essential fatty acid components found in good-quality shea butter and negates the therapeutic properties of essential fatty acids. Thus, shea butter must be produced so that its natural antioxidants remain intact. These antioxidants include vitamin E (tocopherol), which not only heals the skin but helps to prevent oxidation of the butter's essential fatty acids.

High-performance liquid chromatography of the tocopherol content of shea butters from different regions of Africa report great differences among different areas. The effect of an area's environmental stress, climate, and heat are largely responsible for varying levels of alpha-tocopherol levels.[4] In 102 different shea butter samples from 11 countries, the total tocopherol content (which includes the alpha, beta, gamma, and delta forms of tocopherol) ranged from 29 to 809 mg of shea butter, with a mean average of 220 mg/g.

Alpha-tocopherol, the most prevalent form of vitamin E in the samples, accounted for an average of 64% of the total tocopherol content. Shea butters from shea trees situated in hot, dry climates had the highest levels of alpha-tocopherol. For example, in samples from N'Djamena, Chad-which is one of the hottest areas in Africa-the mean average was 414 mg/g. Concentrations of alpha-tocopherol were lowest in samples from the cool highland areas of northern Uganda, with an average of 29 mg/g.

Chapter 6
Modern Use in the Western World

In Germany, shea butter products were first imported at the end of the 19th century. As early as 1940, many scientists verified earlier observations that, among the populations using shea butter, skin diseases were rare and the skin was exceptionally supple and smooth.

The first large-scale clinical tests of shea butter in skin care were performed between 1930 and 1952. Even then, chemists were intrigued by the high fat content of the seeds and the butter's stability without any added preservatives. In the mid-1960s, shea butter all but disappeared from world markets and was supplanted by cocoa butter and cocoa-based products promoted by and used extensively throughout the industrial countries of the West. The main reason was cost in terms of supply and demand. At that time cocoa was much easier to obtain and extract than shea. Hence, despite the fact that shea is more effective than cocoa butter, the popularity of the latter grew instead.[5]

In recent years, however, Western consumers have begun to favor quality over quantity and convenience. Shea has regained significance and popularity as a clinically proven nourishing moisturizer, either in its own right or as a component of high-quality cosmetics and toiletries. Some firms that regularly use shea butter include The Body Shop, Estee Lauder, Crabtree & Evelyn, Smith & Hawken, and Bare Escentuals. A French perfume company, L'Occitane, has developed an entire line of cosmetics based on shea butter. Revlon, the Bobbi Brown line of cosmetics, and the Unilever Corporation all use shea butter in numerous products sold around the world.

Aside from its topical skin applications, shea is used in a host of everyday goods. Such products include candles, soap, massage lotions, animal feed, margarine, cakes, and a wide variety of confections and candy.[5, 6]

Surprisingly, shea is a primary ingredient of that most delicious of all candies, chocolate. Shea is used throughout the world as a cocoa butter substitute in chocolate production. Declining cocoa tree populations have made shea butter much less expensive than cocoa butter, and thus shea makes chocolate more affordable, which increases chocolate sales. Shea butter has a lower melting point than cocoa butter, making it easier to work with.[7] It is mostly used by mass manufacturers of low- to mid-priced chocolates. Firms such as the Mars Corporation, Cadbury, and the Swiss firm Lindt all use this cocoa butter substitute.

Chapter 7
Comparison of Shea Butter to Other Oils and Emollients

Most seed oils can be divided into two important fractions.
The first fraction is the called the saponifiable fraction, which
contains most of shea's moisturizing properties. This is the
moisturizing fraction. The second fraction is called the
nonsaponifiable fraction, which contains most of the healing
properties-the healing fraction.

What sets shea butter apart from other seed oils is its
exceptionally large healing fraction. The healing fraction
contains important nutrients, vitamins, and other valuable
phytonutrients that make shea therapeutic. Depending on the
source, the size of the healing fraction may range from 5%
and upward. Some report the healing fraction as high as 17%.
The larger the healing fraction, the better the chances of a
good-quality shea butter.

In other seed oils, the healing fraction is very small, often in
the range of 1% or less. While other seed oils may have a
good to excellent moisturizing fraction, these oils contain little
or no healing fraction. Because shea butter has such a large
healing fraction, in addition to its moisturizing fraction,
regular use of this natural cream can treat many skin problems

including blemishes, wrinkles, itching, sunburns, small skin wounds, eczema, skin allergies, insect bites, frost bite, and other skin conditions. These unique healing properties result in the shea tree being called the *karite* tree, which means "Tree of Life."

The moisturizers in shea butter are the same ones produced by the sebaceous glands in the skin. Since shea butter mimics the effects of these naturally produced moisturizers that the skin itself produces, it is no wonder that shea butter is such a superior moisturizer and protectant. The positive biochemical and physiological effect of shea butter on skin injuries makes this cream ideal for wound healing. Many users of shea butter report that shea butter promotes and accelerates wound healing and has anti-aging properties. Shea acts as an antioxidant and exerts a positive effect by increasing the skin's microcirculation of blood. Shea's superiority becomes clear in a comparison with other nut butters and oils.

Cocoa Butter

Cocoa butter is obtained from the fruit of the Cacao tree (*Theobroma cacao*), which grows in the world's tropical regions. The butter is extracted from the seed kernels and is further refined and deodorized to yield a tan, nearly odorless butter. It is a relatively hard butter with a steep melting curve that is ideal for body care products. Cocoa butter is used in a variety of cosmetic, toiletry, and pharmaceutical applications to reduce dry skin and improve skin elasticity while imparting a natural color and relatively little odor. Cocoa butter does a credible job of moisturizing, but unlike shea butter, it has no demonstrable or inherent healing properties.

Hemp Seed Oil

Hemp seed butter is produced from the oil of expeller-pressed seeds of the hemp plant (*Cannabis sativa*) and then is mixed with varying amounts of hydrogenated oils. Hemp seed oil is used in cosmetics and toiletries because of its high content of essential fatty acids. Hemp seed butter is produced using the fatty fractions and unsaponifiables (natural waxes and paraffins) that are collected during the refining process before being blended with hydrogenated vegetable (hemp seed) oil to produce a butter-like material suitable for use in cosmetics and toiletries.

Just as the regular ingestion of hydrogenated oils is unhealthy, so to is their continued use in skin products. These oils are needed to make some nut oils thicker, creamier, or more ointment-like for easier use but contribute nothing to health benefits. Unsaponifiables are the not-so-desirable fractions that coat the skin rather than promote healing.

Hemp seed oil feels relatively dry yet provides excellent lubricity without being greasy. Curiously, hemp seed oil is illegal to manufacture in the United States, where it is against the law to grow the plant even for oil production or other manufacturing purposes such as fiber manufacturing. The lawmakers of today may have forgotten that George Washington himself grew this valuable plant as a source of fiber for rope.

Illipe Tree Butter

The Illipe tree (*Shorea stenoptera*) is a magnificent tree that grows in the forests of Borneo in the South Pacific. Illipe butter appears light tan and has long-lasting moisturizing properties. It is most renowned as a skin softener. Illipe closely resembles cocoa butter chemically, yet it has a higher melting point, making it ideal for use in bar soaps, lip balms, lipsticks, and other stick-type applications.

Kokum Tree Butter

Kokum butter is obtained from the fruit of the Kokum (*Garcinia indica*) or "Kokam" tree grown in the central east region of India. The butter is extracted from its fruit kernels and further processed and refined to yield a very white butter with a fairly mild odor, a butter suitable for cosmetics and toiletries. Kokum butter exhibits excellent emollient properties and high oxidative stability, which can improve emulsion integrity. With its relatively higher melt point, Kokum butter melts slightly at skin temperatures, making it ideal for lipsticks and balms; the butter is also a great addition to bar soaps and skin lotions.

Macadamia Nut Butter

Macadamia seed butter is obtained by cold pressing the nuts (seeds) of the *Macadamia ternifolia* tree, followed by a full refining process to render a light-colored oil with a mild odor. The natural oil contains essential fatty acids but also contains unsaponifiables, which are collected during the refining and deodorization process and are blended with hydrogenated macadamia seed oil to render a butter-like consistency suitable for personal care products.

Macadamia seed butter has exceptional emollience and lubricity yet allows good skin penetration. As is the case with most of these other butters and oils, macadamia nut butter is much less desirable for regular use because it is expensive, is commonly adulterated with hydrogenated oils or fats, and has more naturally occurring paraffins or waxes.

Chapter 8
Scientific Research and Validation

Major Constituents of Shea Butter
Shea butter contains numerous compounds, but the most important fractions are essential fatty acids, saponins, and triterpenes. Shea butter includes high levels of UV-absorbing triterpene esters made of:

- Cinnamic acid
- Tocopherols (vitamin E)
- Hytosterols

These compounds help shea butter heal and protect the skin from sunburn and imbue the butter with antioxidant properties allowing for long-term stability during storage. In particular, the copious unsaponifiable fats within shea are natural components of human skin and precursors to cholesterol and other sterols, which explains shea's powerful ability to bind moisture within the outer skin layer. This binding ability helps the skin to retain its suppleness and elasticity.

Shea butter contains 11% unsaponifiable fats or oils compared to the 1. 2 % found in olive oil and 1.5% found in sesame oil. Unsaponifiables are a large group of compounds called *plant steroids* or *sterolins*. They soften the skin, provide superior moisture to the upper layer of the skin, and reduce scars. Good shea butter is expeller-pressed without solvents, making a lipid suitable for soaps, cosmetics, and toiletries. Such butter melts at skin temperatures, making it ideal for lip and body balms as well as bar soaps and lotions. Shea butter is renowned for its skin softening and its moisture retention. This high percentage of unsaponifiables consists of such components as phytosterols and includes various fractions such as:

- Campesterol
- Stigmasterol
- Beta-sitosterol
- Alpha-spinosterol

Shea butter also contains triterpenes such as:

- Cinnamic acid esters
- Alpha- and beta-amyrin
- Parkeol
- Buytospermol
- Lupeol

Hydrocarbons such as karitene also are found in small amounts.[8, 9]

Shea butter is composed of five principal essential fatty acids.[10]

- Palmitic
- Stearic
- Oleic
- Linoleic
- Arachidic

Some 85% to 90% of the fatty acids in shea butter are stearic and oleic acids.[10] The relative proportions of these two fatty acids produce differences in the consistency of shea butter. Its solid consistency is due to large amounts of stearic acid; the percentage of oleic acid influences how soft or hard the shea butter is.

Chevreul (1823) first described stearic acid while researching fats. It is the highest-molecular-weight saturated fatty acid and is abundant in fats and oils. Seeds and marine oils contain small amounts of stearic acid. Milk fats (5% to 15%), lard (10%), tallow (15% to 30%), and cocoa and shea butters (30% to 35%) are the richest sources of stearic acid. The acid is the principal constituent of hydrogenated fats and oils (accounting for ~90%).

The proportions of stearic and oleic acids in the shea kernels and butter differ across the distribution range of the species.

Ugandan shea butter has consistently high oleic acid content and is liquid at warm ambient temperatures. Ugandan shea butter fractionates into liquid and solid phases, and it is the source of liquid shea oil. The fatty acid proportion of West African shea butter varies much more widely than Ugandan shea butter: the oleic content ranges from 37% to 55%. Variability can even be high in relatively small local populations. A tree that produces hard butter can be right next to one that produces soft butter.

Nuts are gathered from a wide area for local production, so the consistency of shea butter is determined by the average fatty acid profile of the total tree population. A study[10] showed that within West Africa, the average stearic acid content is higher in shea butter from the Mossi plateau region of Burkina Faso; this butter was harder than shea butter from other West African regions. This study also found that the overall concentration and relative phenolic content in shea kernels varied regionally. The authors hypothesized that the overall concentration of phenols in shea kernels is linked to the amount of environmental stress each tree endures. Through their moisture-binding properties, the unsaponifiable fatty components are particularly responsible how shea butter makes the skin feel soft and smooth. Triterpenic alcohols and the cinnamon esters within shea provide important natural protection from ultraviolet sunlight rays (wavelength = 275 nm), which help explain this product's skin-protective and anti-aging properties.

The vitamin E, vitamin A, and allantoin within shea butter protects the skin from drying out and aging; it also acts as an anti-inflammatory agent and antioxidants. The allantoin and phytosterols in shea are likely to be responsible for the promotion of cellular growth; the resinous esters help to heal the skin and wounds. Kariten, a blend of various derivatives with pro-vitamin properties, may also be a factor in healing and probably helps to nourish skin cells.

A 2003 study [11] characterized and quantified the most important phenolic compounds in shea butter, eight of which are catechins (also found in green tea). The phenolic profile is similar to that of green olive oil. Unfortunately, this study of phenolic compounds tested shea butter that had been extracted with hexane. The authors note the likelihood that this more-modern extraction process altered or reduced the beneficial chemical compounds, the levels of which would be much higher in traditionally extracted shea butter. Furthermore, the authors noted that the catechin content of shea butter approaches that of ripe olives.

As mentioned previously, shea butter contains the ingredient cinnamic acid, a substance very closely related to the cinnamon found in one's kitchen cabinet. The cinnamic acid in shea butter is mainly bound to other ingredients; however, as shea butter loses its natural integrity, the amount of bound cinnamic acid decreases and the amount of free or unbound cinnamic acid increases. The lower the amount of bound cinnamic acid in shea butter, the lower its effectiveness in healing. However, shea butter that has lost its natural integrity (i.e., oxidized or degraded shea butter) still retains its moisturizing ability but can no longer heal many skin conditions. This means that products containing poor-quality shea butter have the same characteristics of more common oils or fats-good for moisturizing but not for healing.

Human Studies

A clinical study undertaken by Poelman and associates [12] in France (where shea remains a popular moisturizer) demonstrates the butter's effects. Ofin, a cream containing 5% shea butter, and a placebo cream (control) were applied at the beginning of the 30-day experiment and reapplied daily to the forearm of 10 volunteers.

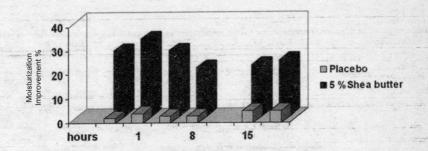

An average of ten skin conductimetric measures were calculated to detect differences between shea-treated and untreated skin. As the above graph shows, moisture improvement was ten times better in the shea-treated skin than in placebo-treated skin.

These tests showed that shea application resulted in short-term moisturizing of the skin. This effect peaked after one hour and persisted for an average of eight hours. In all subjects, a single daily application of shea butter maintained very good moisturizing of the skin's superficial layers.

In a French Ph.D. thesis, F. Renard describes two clinical studies.[13] The research group performed the first study on 30 volunteers, ages 29 to 82 years. Shea butter was applied via daily massage as a balm for 4 to 8 months to determine its impact on several parameters of skin condition. The results, summarized in the graph below, demonstrated major improvements in various skin conditions.

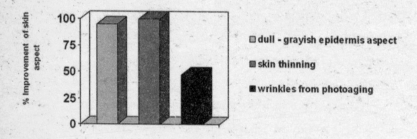

First, dull, grayish complexion tones were eliminated and replaced by smoother, brighter, clearer skin within a few weeks. Second, skin thinning was apparently minimized: skin texture became fuller and the skin's appearance improved. This regenerating effect is likely due to (1) the action of the unsaponifiable lipids within shea butter and (2) the active components known to reactivate collagen synthesis. Finally, the trial demonstrated that wrinkles caused by prolonged sun exposure (a process called photo aging) were visibly diminished in half of the study volunteers.

The second study by this same group was designed to determine the effects of shea butter on dry, delicate, or aging skin. Forty-nine volunteers applied either 15% or pure shea formula to their skin twice daily.

The results were similar for both formulas, suggesting that the 15% formula is already "saturated"-that is, it contains as many shea ingredients as can be active within and upon the outer layers of the skin.

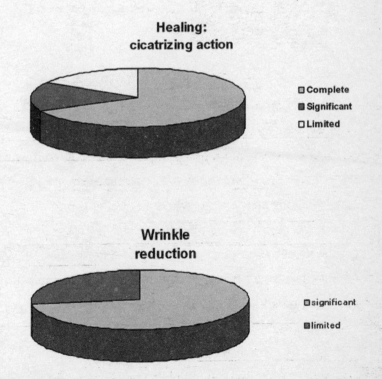

Healing: cicatrizing action

- Complete
- Significant
- Limited

Wrinkle reduction

- significant
- limited

As the previous charts show, shea application clearly produced a healing (cicatrizing) effect on hand dermatitis, sunburns, and scars in 70% of those tested. Wrinkles were reduced and skin suppleness improved in 75% of volunteers.

So how does shea butter bring about these dramatic effects? Our current understanding suggests that the active components of shea butter promote wound healing and minimize scarring and burns by accelerating the regeneration of skin cells. Shea butter also promotes blood flow to the skin's outer layers, supplying the cells therein with the oxygen, growth factors, immune cells, and other nourishing factors responsible for a toned and healthy glow.

Shea butter's role in promoting blood flow has been confirmed by a recent human clinical study[13] that tested shea butter's anti-inflammatory and healing effects in 33 volunteers affected by rhinitis, a chronic inflammatory condition associated with moderate to severe nasal congestion. Nasal congestion is caused by swollen internal nasal tissues (edema) that can be relieved in two ways: by treating the symptom with vasoconstrictors, which reduce fluid influx within the tissues, or by treating the cause with an anti-inflammatory agent, which inhibits the swelling process from the outset. (Shea butter falls into the latter category.) The outcome of this study, summarized in the graphic plot below, confirmed anecdotal reports that patients who applied shea butter to the affected area experienced greater relief than patients who were given a standard decongestant drug (xylometazoline) or placebo (white petroleum jelly). These results strongly suggest that shea is a highly effective, natural nasal anti-inflammatory and decongestant.[14]

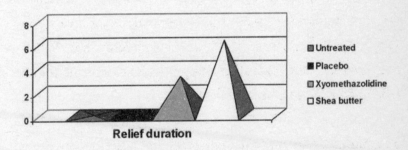

Relief duration

Fats derived from shea seeds are exceptionally versatile and have many uses outside of the cosmetic realm. Shea is also used as a food, for lamp fuel, and as an insulating material for housing. Shea oleine, an oil fraction also derived from the shea nut, is used widely throughout Nigeria and other African countries as a frying oil and, after hardening, in margarine and toffee fat. In its Central African homeland, the shea tree is also the main source of fat for cooking. One also can eat the fruits containing the seeds or nuts that produce shea oil.

Studies are under way in the West to ascertain whether shea-derived oils may improve our daily diet. Shea seeds contain particularly high amounts (~42%) of the saturated dietary fat stearic acid. One study[15] tested shea nut oil supplementation (shea oil or fats derived from other seeds) in 15 men for 3 weeks. Shea nut oil supplementation significantly reduced plasma cholesterol (22%), LDL cholesterol (26%), apolipoprotein B (18%), HDL cholesterol (12%), apolipoprotein A-I (13%), and factor VII coagulant activity (13%; $P = .001$).

A crossover study[16] involving ten middle-aged men tested the effects of a 20-day "stabilization diet" followed by two 40-day "intervention diets" to determine the cholesterolemic effect of high amounts of stearic acid in a natural diet. The subjects consumed a 20-day stabilization diet followed by two 40-day intervention diets containing either 1.5% of energy as stearic acid and 7.3% of energy as palmitic acid (16:0)-the low-stearate diet-or 7.3% of energy as stearic acid and 2.4% of energy as palmitic acid-the high-stearate diet. The experimental diets also contained approximately 10% of energy each as saturated and monounsaturated fatty acids and 7.2%-8% of energy as polyunsaturated fatty acids. The primary source of stearic acid was shea nut oil (also known as shea butter) in the high-stearate diet and palm oil and butter in the low-stearate diet. Plasma total, low-density-lipoprotein, and high-density lipoprotein cholesterol were significantly lower with the high-stearate than with the low-stearate diet. Total fecal fatty acid excretion was higher throughout the high-stearate period. Apparent digestibility of the major dietary fatty acids showed that all of the selected fatty acids, except stearic acid, were at least 95% absorbed.

These data demonstrate that diets containing about two times the usual amount of stearic acid consumed in the United States contributed to an increase in plasma lipoprotein concentrations at 40 d from an earlier decrease at 20 d. The time required to achieve stable cholesterol concentrations appears to vary with the type of saturated fatty acid.

The end result is that high levels of fats derived from shea butter are easily digested and excreted but can lead to higher lipid levels if used on an ongoing basis, as would be expected with any high-fat diet.

A randomized, cross-over study of cholesterol in healthy young men reported some interesting findings.[17] Ten young healthy men were served two meals (1.2 g fat/kg body weight) containing fat enriched with either stearic acid (shea butter) or myristic acid (produced by inter-esterification). The meals were given in the morning after 12 h of fasting and again after 8 h (in the afternoon). The different meals were given at different days separated by a washout period. Blood samples were taken before and 2, 4, 6, 8, and 24 h after the first meal.

The results show that intake of individual dietary SFA (saturated fatty acids) may affect fasting HDL cholesterol within 24 h: after this short period, the HDL cholesterol concentration was higher after meals containing myristic acid than after meals containing stearic acid (shea). Myristic acid resulted in a higher increase in postprandial HDL levels. Shea butter also had much less of an effect on blood cholesterol than fats containing higher levels of myristic acid over the study's time frame.

The Danish company Aarhus United has already applied for U.S. New Dietary Supplement Notification status for their cholesterol-lowering product, SheaNature. In clinical tests[18] at the University of Aalborg, this patented shea butter extract reduced blood cholesterol levels by 10% to 15%. SheaNature and other shea-based dietary supplements may be an appealing natural alternative to traditional cholesterol-lowering drugs. Studies conducted thus far have shown no side effects with these supplements; furthermore, toxicological studies prove that shea extract is completely safe for human consumption.

One of shea butter's particularly interesting properties is that it binds heavy metals in the body, enabling the system to excrete them before they are absorbed. This trait is highly interesting to people who live in areas of significant water pollution, where increased concentrations of heavy metals contribute to high rates of chronic disease. This is a greater problem than is realized even in developed countries-including major population centers with modern water treatment facilities.[19]

A French study[20] reported that shea butter was better for ointments than two of the most commonly used gels, Vaseline and lanoline. The researchers discovered that shea butter released the active ingredient suspended in the ointment, in this case an antibiotic, faster and more completely than the other ointment bases.

Animal Studies
Researchers often use rats to determine whether a product is toxic or produces other negative symptoms at high doses. One such rat study[21] tested the effects of huge amounts of shea butter (hardened oleine)-greater than 7.5 g/kg of body weight per day-and found zero negative effects.

Furthermore, these absurd amounts of shea butter had none of the negative effects on reproduction (reduced pregnancy or birth rates) that are common with high-fat diets. In other words, if there is such a thing as a healthy fat, this is it.

A related rat study,[22] part of a series, compared the carcinogenic potential of 15% shea oleine with 15% shea nut oil and palm oil following 104 weeks of dietary administration. The study evaluated mortality, clinical signs, body weight, food intake, clinical disease, organ weights, and macroscopic and histopathological (cellular) examination in addition to tumor type and incidence. Results showed that shea oleine produced no adverse effects and had zero tumorigenic (cancer-creating) potential. Shea oleine showed no tumorigenic signs even following dietary administration at a rate of 7.5 g/kg of body weight per day.

Even tests of the smallest fractions found in shea nuts-the coloring of the nut itself, which is used in food dyes-have yielded good results.[23] Rats fed large amounts of just the dye derived from shea nuts exhibited no symptoms of toxicity whatsoever.

According to another rat study,[24] even a diet composed mostly of fats from shea butter causes no weight gain. In fact, the subjects experienced a small but definite weight loss!

Chapter 9
Skin Products and Effects

Who among us doesn't use moisturizers to fight dry skin? We face a bewildering array of crèmes, lotions, and oils for the face, for the hands, and for the body. These products seem to become increasingly "high-tech" and, some might say, synthetic in their composition. As these products become more complex, so do manufacturers' promises of what these preparations deliver.

A better solution to skin care might be to turn back the clock away from synthetic formulas to harness the benefits of a purely natural moisturizer. After all, centuries of satisfied, youthful-looking women (and men) can't be wrong! Now that the secret of how shea butter naturally moisturizes, heals, and protects the skin has left Africa and reached the Western world, shea-based products are becoming widely available in many formulas. You may already be using shea butter and not even know it. Many popular, widely used luxury household toiletry products contain shea butter, especially products that are widely marketed in Europe. These products include crèmes, lotions, soaps, massage oils, shower gels, body washes, shampoos and conditioners, sun tan lotions and sun screens, after-sun lotions, make-up, lipsticks, and lip balms. Brands such as Palmolive, Dove, the Boots Spa range, and the Covent Garden-based Sanctuary range all contain shea pearls. These pearls are capsules that dissolve to provide a readily absorbed source of moisture and contain as much as 10% unrefined shea, bound in gelatin or gum Arabic. One of the biggest producers of these capsules is the Swiss company, IMPGA GmbH.

All moisturizers employ the same principle: fats (lipids) in the moisturizer are absorbed by the outer layers of the skin to form a barrier that prevents moisture loss, keeping our skin softer and more supple. Such products are called emollients-products that provide passive protection to the skin rather than delivering any active benefits. Emollients were discussed earlier in the comparisons of various oils and plant butters. Vitamins, minerals, or antioxidants, whether present naturally or later added to a product, may also improve skin health, appearance, and tone; however, whether these additional components actually produce benefits above those delivered by the lipid content of moisturizers remains highly controversial.

So with this vast array of products, how is shea butter different? Is shea butter merely another emollient, or does it contain additional active ingredients than provide extra benefit for the skin? The answer, gained from millennia of historical knowledge and, more recently, from clinical studies, is that shea is so much more than an emollient. The lipid content of unrefined shea butter goes beyond the simple formation of a barrier against moisture loss; it also provides anti-inflammatory support for skin cells and promotes their regeneration. Shea also provides soothing protection against infection and irritation as it supplies damaged skin with crucial nourishing lipids.

Shea butter is available in unrefined or refined form, in unperfumed and uncolored preparations, as a crushed shea seed butter, or as a paste. These formulations deliver shea in its purist and most potent form. Importantly, unrefined, unperfumed shea butter has yet to be associated with any allergies or reactions. Fragranced or colored variations of shea may cause irritation if they happen to contain compounds that "don't agree" with your particular skin type.

Choose your supplier carefully and always read the label. In addition, if you haven't used one of these products before, it is always advisable to do a small skin patch test on a preferred "secluded" region to rule out the possibility of irritation. To avoid such problems, the safest bet is to opt for unperfumed, uncolored shea butter or shea-based products.

Shea-based products tend to fall into two categories: those containing 5% shea butter and those containing 10% or more. Products in the latter category will obviously have more of an effect, delivering greater moisturization. As the studies described earlier show, products containing at least 15% shea butter may be as effective as pure shea butter in delivering certain benefits to skin quality and appearance.

For the best and fastest results to smoother, supple, more nourished and younger-looking skin, shea butter or shea-containing products should be applied generously to the face, hands, and entire body as a daily moisturizer. For treating dry-skin conditions such as eczema, psoriasis, and chapped or chafed skin, apply the butter directly to affected areas of skin.

Chapter 10
Safety/Contraindications

No toxic reactions have ever been noted with shea butter, whether it was used externally or internally. Shea is one of the few natural products that is safe to use even in very large doses. Other seeds and nuts typically used in oil production are associated with molds or aflatoxins (poisons) resulting from molds. Tests show that shea nuts have very few problems in this area, even when the oils are made from discarded or substandard nut stocks.[25]

Chapter 11

Allergic Reactions

No allergies have been noted or reported.

Chapter 12
Who Should Use Shea Butter?

In a word, everyone!

Shea butter and its by-products are one of the richest sources of stearic acid, the beneficial dietary fat. We have seen how preliminary tests demonstrate the effectiveness of this shea-derived oil with a host of ailments, both internal and external-including elevated blood cholesterol levels. Shea butter is an amazing natural moisturizer with excellent soothing, healing, anti-aging, and anti-inflammatory properties. There is nothing on the market quite like shea, which outperforms related products such as cocoa butter in improving skin appearance and quality.

As a skin care product, shea butter comes in many forms and from a wealth of sources and suppliers. You can choose the pure, unrefined forms of shea butter or opt for products that contain 10% to 15% shea. It is best to use high-quality products that contain at least 15% shea butter and to apply them liberally to the face, body, and hands each day; such use will make your skin more supple, firm and yet softer to the touch, brighter, and more youthful.

As the ozone layer degrades, air becomes more polluted, and our diets become less healthy and lower in the good fats and oils so essential to health in general and to the skin specifically, research into the effects of shea butter provides a ray of hope in a sometimes dark world. The hype concerning skin care products continues to grow, and yet few facts or research ever seem to back up the often outlandish claims. With skin cancer rates climbing every year, it is wonderful to know of a product that can help protect us while beautifying, healing, and reducing the signs of aging-and can do it all without bankrupting us. There is a saying that may be appropriate here: "For every disease that we know, God allows a plant to grow."

To put it succinctly: Shea butter is one of the most versatile, safe, and effective botanical extracts on the market today.

References

1. *Travels in the Interior Districts of Africa: performed in the years 1795, 1796, and 1797. With an account of a subsequent mission to that country in 1805.* Ed. J. Whishaw. London, John Murray, 1817.

2. Leach A, McArdle TF, Banya WA, et al. 1999. *Neonatal mortality in a rural area of The Gambia.* Ann Trop Paediatr 19:33-43.

3. Sylla M, Konan L, Doannio JM, Traore S. 2003. *Evaluation of the efficacy of coconut (Cocos nucifera), palm nut (Eleais guineensis) and gobi (Carapa procera) lotions and creams in individual protection against Simulium damnosum s.l. bites in Cote d'Ivoire.* Bull Soc Pathol Exot 96:104-109.

4. Maranz S, Wiesman Z. 2004. *Influence of climate on the tocopherol content of shea butter.* The Phyto-Oleochemical Laboratory, The Institutes for Applied Research, Ben-Gurion University of the Negev, P.O. Box 653, Beer-Sheva, Israel. J Agric Food Chem 52:2934-2937.

5. Irvine F. 1966. *Woody Plants of Ghana: With Special Reference to Their Uses.* London: Oxford University.

6. Mcfee A. 1926. *The Economic Revolution in British West Africa.* London: Routledge.

7. Spangenberg JE, Dionisi F. 2001. *Characterization of cocoa butter and cocoa butter equivalents by bulk and molecular carbon isotope analyses: implications for vegetable fat quantification in chocolate.* J Agric Food Chem 49:4271-4277.

8. Wiesman Z, Marans S, Bianchi G, Bisgaard J. 2003. *Chemical analysis of fruits of Vitellaria paradoxa.* In: Teklehaimanot, Z (ed). *Improved Management of Agroforestry Parkland Systems in Sub-Saharan Africa, Final Report.* Bangor, U.K.: School of Agricultural and Forest Sciences, University of Wales, pp 131-139.

9. Badifu GIO. 1989. *Lipid composition of Nigerian Butyrospermum paradoxum kernel.* J Food Compos Anal 2:238-244.

10. Maranz S, Wiesman Z, Bisgaard J, Bianchi G. 2004. *Germplasm resources of Vitellaria paradoxa based on variations in fat composition across the species distribution range.* Agroforestry Systems 60:71-76.

11. Maranz S, Wiesman Z, Garti N. 2003. *Phenolic constituents of shea (Vitellaria paradoxa) kernels.* J Agric Food Chem 51:6268-6273.

12. Poelman R. 1998. *Les Nouvelles Dermatologiques* 7:78-79. www.nouvellesdermatologiques.com.

13. Renard F. 1990. *Le buerrede karite. Thése de Doctorat en Pharmacie.* UFR de sciences pharmacuetiques. soutenue le 21 decembre 1990, Universite de Bordeaux II, p 100.

14. Tella A. 1979. *Preliminary studies on nasal decongestant activity from the seed of the Shea butter tree, Butyrospermum parkii.* Br J Clin Pharmacol 7:495-497.

15. Tholstrup T, Marckmann P, Jespersen J, Sandstrom B. 1994. F*at high in stearic acid favorably affects blood lipids and factor VII coagulant activity in comparison with fats high in palmitic acid or high in myristic and lauric acids.* Am J Clin Nutr 59:371-377.

16. Dougherty RM, Allman MA, Iacono JM. 1995. *Effects of diets containing high or low amounts of stearic acid on plasma lipoprotein fractions and fecal fatty acid excretion of men.* Am J Clin Nutr 61:1120-1128.

17. Tholstrup T, Vessby B, Sandstrom B. 2003. *Difference in effect of myristic and stearic acid on plasma HDL cholesterol within 24 h in young men.* Eur J Clin Nutr 57:735-742.

18. Eric Berg Schmidt, et al. *Shea nut oil as a lipid lowering drug. The effect of shea nut oil on serumlipids and lipoproteins in normocholesterolemic and mildly hypercholesterolemic humans.* Department of Clinical Biochemistry, Aalborg Hospital, Denmark.

19. Eromosele IC, Otitolaye OO. 1994. *Binding of iron, zinc, and lead ions from aqueous solution by shea butter (Butyrospermun parkii) seed husks.* Bull Environ Contam Toxicol 52:530-537.

20. Thioune O, Khouma B, Diarra M, et al. 2003. *The excipient properties of shea butter compared with vaseline and lanolin.* Laboratoire de Pharmacie Galenique et Legislation, Faculte de Medecine, de Pharmacie et d'Odonto-stomatologie-UCAD, Dakar, Senegal. Pharm Belg 58:81-84.

21. Baldrick P, Robinson JA, Hepburn PA. 2001. *Reproduction studies in the rat with shea oleine and hardened shea oleine.* Consultancy & Regulatory Services, Covance Laboratories Ltd, Otley Road, North Yorkshire HG3 1PY, Harrogate, UK. Food Chem Toxicol 39:923-930.

22. Carthew P, Baldrick P, Hepburn PA. 2001. *An assessment of the carcinogenic potential of shea oleine in the rat.* Safety & Environmental Assurance Centre, Unilever Research, Colworth House, Sharnbrook, Bedfordshire MK41 6EP, United Kingdom. Food Chem Toxicol 39:807-815.

23. Kitamura Y, Nishikawa A, Furukawa F, et al. 2003. *A subchronic toxicity study of shea nut color in Wistar rats.* Division of Pathology, National Institute of Health Sciences, 1-18-1 Kamiyoga, Setagaya-ku, Tokyo 158-8501, Japan. Food Chem Toxicol 41:1537-1542.

24. Earl LK, Baldrick P, Hepburn PA. 2002. *A 13-week feeding study in the rat with shea oleine and hardened shea oleine.* Safety and Environmental Assurance Centre, Unilever Colworth Laboratory, Sharnbrook, Bedfordshire, United Kingdom. Int J Toxicol 21:13-22.

25. Kershaw SJ. 1982. *Occurrence of aflatoxins in oilseeds providing cocoa-butter substitutes.* Appl Environ Microbiol 43:1210-1212

NOTES

NOTES